DEFEATING MEASLES IN CHILDREN

A Parent's Handbook to Recognizing the Culprit Behind Measles, Prevention Strategies, Bathing Technique, Fostering Immunity, and Advocating for Children's Health

Sophia Hawthorne

Table of Contents

Introduction: Importance of Measles Awareness in Children's Health

Childhood is a time of growth, discovery, and boundless potential. It is a phase when children should be free to explore the world, learn, and develop without the threat of preventable diseases casting a shadow over their well-being. Measles, a highly contagious and potentially severe viral infection, stands as a stark reminder of the importance of awareness and preventive measures in safeguarding the health of our youngest generation.

Definition and Impact

Measles, caused by the morbillivirus, can have a profound impact on a child's health. The virus manifests through a combination of symptoms, beginning with a high fever, tiredness, a distinctive barky cough, red or bloodshot eyes, and a runny nose. The ensuing red, blotchy rash can cover the entire body, marking the progression of the disease. Beyond the discomfort of these symptoms lies the potential for severe complications, especially in vulnerable populations such as infants, pregnant individuals, and those with weakened immune systems.

Historical Context

Before the widespread availability of vaccines, measles was a pervasive and life-threatening concern. Hundreds of lives were claimed annually by this once-unchecked virus. The development and distribution of vaccines, particularly the MMR (measles, mumps, rubella) vaccine, marked a turning point in the battle against measles, offering a shield of immunity to countless children.

In the modern era, where vaccination is readily accessible, the importance of measles awareness lies not only in recognizing its symptoms and consequences but also in championing preventive measures that can spare children from unnecessary suffering.

Spread of Measles in Children

Measles spreads rapidly among children, primarily through airborne transmission. In crowded environments like schools, daycare centers, and playgroups, where close contact is inevitable, the virus finds ample opportunities to infect unvaccinated children. The contagious period, starting a few days before the rash appears and lasting several days afterward, poses a significant risk in these communal settings. Awareness of how measles spreads among children is crucial for implementing preventive strategies and protecting our communities.

The introduction serves as a call to action, emphasizing the collective responsibility to raise awareness about measles and its impact on children's health. It urges parents, caregivers, educators, and healthcare providers to join forces in promoting vaccination, dispelling myths, and fostering an environment that prioritizes the well-being of the younger generation.

By understanding the historical context of measles, acknowledging its potential complications, and recognizing the modes of transmission among children, we empower ourselves to take proactive measures. Through education, advocacy, and vaccination, we can create a shield of immunity that guards our little ones against the threat of measles.

Chapter 1: Understanding Measles in Children

Measles, scientifically known as *rubeola*, is a respiratory disease caused by the morbillivirus. It is part of the Paramyxoviridae family and is characterized by a high fever, distinctive skin rash, and respiratory symptoms. The classification of measles involves distinguishing between different strains of the virus and understanding its modes of transmission. Measles, a highly contagious viral infection, has long been a concern in child health, leaving a significant impact on communities worldwide.

There are various strains of morbillivirus, and they can cause different types of measles. While the basic symptoms remain consistent, the severity of the disease can vary. Understanding the nuances of measles classification is crucial for healthcare professionals in diagnosing and treating affected children effectively.

Impact on Child Health

Measles exerts a profound impact on the health of children, particularly those in vulnerable age groups. The initial symptoms often mimic those of common respiratory infections, with a high fever, cough, and runny nose. However, the distinctive feature of measles is the characteristic red, blotchy rash that spreads across the body.

Beyond the discomfort of the symptoms, measles can lead to severe complications, especially in infants and young children. Respiratory issues, pneumonia, and ear infections are common, and in rare cases, the infection can progress to more severe conditions such as encephalitis. Measles can be particularly challenging for children with weakened immune systems, emphasizing the importance of understanding the impact of this disease on child health.

Before the development and widespread distribution of vaccines, measles was a pervasive and deadly threat, especially among children. In the pre-vaccination era, approximately 400 to 500 deaths occurred each year in the United States due to measles.

The introduction of the measles vaccine, particularly the MMR (measles, mumps, rubella) vaccine, marked a turning point in the battle against this viral adversary. Vaccination campaigns, especially targeting children, significantly reduced the incidence and severity of measles.

Despite the progress made, measles remains a concern globally, especially in regions with lower vaccination rates. The historical context serves as a reminder of the ongoing importance of vaccination efforts and the potential consequences of complacency in the face of preventable diseases.

Chapter 2: Recognizing Measles Symptoms in Children

Early Symptoms and Warning Signs

Measles often begins with a deceptive phase, resembling common respiratory infections. However, vigilant parents and caregivers can discern early symptoms that signal a potential measles infection. One of the primary indicators is a high fever, often exceeding 101 degrees Fahrenheit. This initial elevation in body temperature may be accompanied by tiredness, a barky cough, red or bloodshot eyes, and a runny nose.

The challenge lies in distinguishing these early symptoms from those of other viral infections. Measles, however, carries its unique signature, and the combination of a high fever with respiratory symptoms should raise suspicions, particularly in unvaccinated or under-vaccinated children.

Measles Rash: Identification and Characteristics

A few days after the onset of early symptoms, a hallmark feature of measles emerges – the characteristic rash. This red, blotchy rash typically begins on the face before spreading downward to cover the entire body. The progression of the rash is a defining aspect of measles, and its appearance raises the diagnostic certainty.

The rash itself undergoes a distinctive transformation. Initially, flat red spots emerge on the face, which then spread and evolve into smaller raised white spots. The merging of these spots as the rash progresses down the body creates a visually striking manifestation of the disease. Understanding the evolution of the measles rash is pivotal for accurate identification and differentiation from other childhood rashes.

When to Seek Medical Attention

Recognizing measles symptoms is not only about identifying the disease but also about understanding when to seek medical attention. Measles is not a trivial childhood illness, and prompt intervention is crucial to mitigate complications and prevent further spread.

If a child exhibits the early symptoms of measles, especially in regions where the virus is prevalent, seeking medical attention promptly is imperative. Healthcare professionals can conduct diagnostic assessments, including laboratory tests if necessary, to confirm the presence of the virus. Early diagnosis allows for timely intervention, supportive care, and the implementation of preventive measures to protect others in the vicinity.

Moreover, when the characteristic rash appears, it serves as a definitive sign to consult a healthcare provider. The emergence of the rash marks the height of contagiousness, and isolation measures become vital to prevent the spread of the virus within communities.

Parents and caregivers should be vigilant about any signs of respiratory distress, persistent fever, or other concerning symptoms during the course of measles. These may indicate potential

complications that require immediate medical
attention.

Chapter 3: Causes of Measles in Children

Morbillivirus - The Culprit Behind Measles

Measles is caused by the morbillivirus, a member of the Paramyxoviridae family. This enveloped, single-stranded RNA virus is highly contagious and exhibits a remarkable ability to exploit the human respiratory system for its propagation. The morbillivirus primarily targets humans, making it the sole reservoir for this infectious agent.

Upon entering the respiratory tract, typically through inhalation, the morbillivirus finds a hospitable environment for replication. The virus then launches a systematic attack on the host's immune system, subverting its defenses and paving the way for the clinical manifestations of measles.

The journey of morbillivirus infection is a dynamic process, unfolding in stages within the host's body. Initially, the virus gains entry into the respiratory epithelium, where it establishes an initial infection. This marks the beginning of the incubation period, a phase where the virus replicates silently, preparing for the impending assault on the host's immune system.

As the virus multiplies, it enters the bloodstream, facilitating systemic dissemination throughout the body. It is during this viremic phase that early symptoms such as fever, cough, and runny nose emerge, providing the first indications of a measles infection. The morbillivirus, adept at evading the immune response, orchestrates a strategic takeover, leading to the more distinctive signs of measles in the subsequent stages.

The transmission dynamics of morbillivirus play a pivotal role in the epidemiology of measles. Once an individual becomes infected, the virus can be shed into the environment through respiratory secretions, creating a reservoir of contagious particles. Airborne transmission is a hallmark feature of measles, allowing the virus to linger in the air and potentially infect susceptible individuals within the vicinity.

Understanding the morbillivirus as the mastermind behind measles is foundational for implementing preventive measures. Vaccination, which introduces a weakened form of the virus to stimulate the immune system, stands as a powerful defense against this infectious adversary. The exploration of the morbillivirus in this chapter sets the stage for comprehending the nuanced interactions between the virus and its human host, offering insights crucial for devising strategies to thwart the spread of measles among children.

Airborne Transmission and Contagious Period

Measles is categorized as an airborne disease, signifying that the virus can be transmitted through respiratory droplets released into the air by an infected individual. When a person with measles breathes, coughs, sneezes, or talks, tiny particles containing the virus become suspended in the air. These airborne droplets can linger in the environment for up to two hours after the infected person has left the area, posing a risk of exposure to anyone entering that space.

The airborne nature of measles contributes significantly to its rapid spread in crowded places and communal settings. Lack of proper ventilation enhances the persistence of viral particles in the air, creating an environment conducive to transmission. Understanding this mode of transmission emphasizes the importance of preventive measures, especially in places where people gather, such as schools, daycare centers, and public transportation.

Measles exhibits a prolonged contagious period, spanning several days before the onset of the characteristic rash and persisting for about four days afterward. This extended period of infectivity poses challenges for containment efforts. Individuals infected with measles can unknowingly spread the virus during the prodromal phase, when symptoms such as fever, cough, and runny nose are present but the rash has not yet appeared.

The contagious period underscores the need for swift identification and isolation of suspected cases to prevent further transmission. Healthcare providers play a crucial role in recognizing potential measles cases, conducting diagnostic assessments, and implementing isolation measures to protect both the infected individual and those in close proximity.

Common Modes of Measles Spread among Children

Children, with their natural inclination for close contact and shared spaces, are particularly susceptible to measles transmission. Common modes of measles spread among children encompass various scenarios within communal settings:

1. **Close Contact**: Measles spreads efficiently through close contact. Children playing together, sharing toys, or engaging in activities that involve physical proximity provide opportunities for the virus to transfer from one individual to another.

2. **Crowded Environments**: In crowded places like schools, daycare centers, and playgroups, where children gather in significant numbers, the risk of airborne transmission escalates. Poorly ventilated spaces exacerbate the likelihood of exposure.

3. **Schools and Childcare Facilities**: Educational institutions and childcare facilities

serve as hotspots for measles transmission. The combination of a high number of unvaccinated or under-vaccinated children, coupled with shared spaces, creates an environment conducive to the rapid spread of the virus.

4. **Lack of Immunization**: Unvaccinated or under-vaccinated children contribute substantially to the circulation of measles within communities. The absence of immunization not only heightens the risk of infection in individual children but also poses a broader threat to public health.

5. **Transmission from Pregnant Individuals to Babies:** Infants born to mothers with measles during pregnancy can contract the virus either during childbirth or through breastfeeding. This underscores the importance of vaccination for pregnant

individuals to protect both maternal and child health.

Chapter 4: Prevention Strategies for Measles in Children

Importance of Childhood Vaccination

The foundation of preventing measles in children rests upon the bedrock of childhood vaccination. Immunization emerges as a formidable shield, fortifying young ones against the insidious morbillivirus and its potential ravages. The importance of childhood vaccination extends beyond individual protection, creating a communal barricade that curtails the spread of measles within communities.

Childhood vaccination, particularly the Measles, Mumps, Rubella (MMR) vaccine, marks a triumph in preventive medicine.

Administered in two doses during early childhood, the vaccine not only guards against measles but also offers defense against mumps and rubella. This holistic approach maximizes the impact of vaccination, ensuring a comprehensive shield against multiple infectious threats.

The significance of childhood vaccination resonates in the concept of herd immunity, where a sufficiently immunized population forms a collective defense. This concept is particularly crucial for safeguarding those who cannot receive vaccines due to medical reasons. By achieving and maintaining high vaccination coverage, communities create a formidable barrier against measles, enhancing the resilience of society at large.

Public health initiatives underscore the imperative of childhood vaccination, advocating for timely immunization to confer durable protection. Through awareness campaigns, educational programs, and routine vaccination schedules, the goal is to instill a sense of responsibility among parents, caregivers, and communities to prioritize the health and well-being of children.

Vaccine Schedule and Types

The backbone of effective vaccination lies in adherence to a well-defined schedule that optimizes the body's immune response. For measles, mumps, and rubella prevention, the Measles, Mumps, Rubella (MMR) vaccine stands as a beacon. The vaccine schedule is carefully crafted to align with critical developmental milestones in childhood.

The first dose of the MMR vaccine is typically administered around 12-15 months of age, capitalizing on the maturation of the immune system. This initial exposure primes the body to recognize and mount a defense against the viruses. The second dose is then administered at 4-6 years of age, reinforcing and extending the immunity conferred by the first dose. This dual-dose strategy ensures a robust and sustained shield against measles, mumps, and rubella.

The timing of these doses is pivotal. The first dose provides a foundational layer of protection, while the second dose, administered as children enter school, bolsters and extends that protection into adolescence. The meticulous sequencing of vaccine doses is a testament to the precision required in orchestrating a robust defense against infectious threats.

The diversity of vaccine types reflects the nuanced approach to fortifying the immune system against measles. The MMR vaccine, a live attenuated vaccine, takes center stage in the prevention of measles, mumps, and rubella. Live attenuated vaccines contain weakened forms of the viruses, offering a safe yet potent stimulus for the immune system.

The live attenuated nature of the MMR vaccine ensures a comprehensive immune response, including the production of antibodies and the activation of cellular immunity. This multifaceted defense equips the body with the tools needed to recognize and neutralize the viruses upon subsequent exposure. The long-lasting immunity conferred by live attenuated vaccines contributes to the durability of protection against these infectious diseases.

Beyond individual protection, the inclusion of vaccines in national immunization programs reflects a collective commitment to public health. The selection of vaccine types is informed by a careful balance between efficacy, safety, and the ability to confer broad immunity within populations. The ongoing advancements in vaccine research and development continue to refine the arsenal of vaccines, ensuring their adaptability to evolving infectious threats.

Overcoming Vaccine Hesitancy

Vaccine hesitancy is a complex phenomenon influenced by a myriad of factors. Perceptions of vaccine safety, mistrust of healthcare systems, and exposure to misinformation can sow seeds of doubt, creating hesitancy among parents and caregivers. Cultural, religious, and socio-economic considerations further shape individual attitudes towards vaccination.

Addressing vaccine hesitancy requires a nuanced understanding of these diverse factors. It involves recognizing the validity of individual concerns while providing evidence-based information to dispel myths and misconceptions. The human aspect of vaccine hesitancy emphasizes the importance of open and empathetic communication between healthcare providers and communities.

Communication Strategies

Effective communication stands as a linchpin in dismantling barriers to vaccination. Healthcare providers play a pivotal role in engaging with parents and caregivers, offering clear and transparent information about the safety and efficacy of vaccines. This includes explaining the rigorous processes involved in vaccine development, testing, and monitoring.

Public health campaigns, rooted in evidence-based information, contribute to dismantling misconceptions and fostering a culture of vaccination. Leveraging various communication channels, from traditional media to social platforms, helps disseminate accurate information widely. Tailoring communication strategies to diverse cultural and linguistic contexts enhances their effectiveness.

Building Trust

Fostering trust in the healthcare system is paramount in overcoming vaccine hesitancy.

This involves cultivating a collaborative relationship between healthcare providers and communities. Building trust requires acknowledging historical context, addressing disparities in access to healthcare, and actively involving communities in the decision-making processes related to vaccination programs.

The human touch plays a pivotal role in building trust. Personalized interactions, where healthcare providers listen to and address individual concerns, create a foundation for trust. Sharing personal stories and testimonials from individuals who have experienced the positive impact of vaccination can also resonate deeply with hesitant individuals.

Community Engagement

Community engagement stands as a powerful strategy in overcoming vaccine hesitancy.

Mobilizing community leaders, influencers, and trusted figures to advocate for vaccination enhances the credibility of public health messages. Community-driven initiatives, such as town hall meetings, workshops, and forums, provide spaces for open dialogue and address concerns in a collaborative manner.

Chapter 5: Treatment Options for Measles in Children

Antiviral medications represent a class of drugs designed to combat viral infections by either directly inhibiting viral replication or bolstering the host's immune response. In the context of measles, the application of antiviral drugs, particularly Ribavirin, has been explored, albeit cautiously and with careful consideration of specific scenarios.

Ribavirin: Unraveling its Role

Ribavirin is an antiviral medication that has exhibited activity against a range of RNA viruses, including the measles virus. While its use in the routine treatment of uncomplicated measles is not endorsed, Ribavirin may be considered in cases of severe or complicated measles, such as those involving immunocompromised individuals or situations where the infection poses an increased risk of adverse outcomes.

The decision to utilize Ribavirin is made on a case-by-case basis and is typically guided by healthcare providers. It is crucial to emphasize that the routine use of antiviral medications for measles is not universally recommended, and their application remains a subject of ongoing research and evaluation.

Considerations and Limitations

The potential use of antiviral medications prompts a careful weighing of benefits and risks. While these medications may offer some therapeutic value in certain contexts, considerations such as side effects, tolerability, and the overall risk-benefit profile influence their appropriateness in individual cases.

Additionally, the evolving nature of viral infections introduces complexities in antiviral drug development. Measles, as a dynamic RNA virus, can exhibit genetic diversity, potentially impacting the efficacy of antiviral treatments. The adaptability of the virus underscores the importance of ongoing research to refine and tailor treatment strategies.

Guidance and Supervision

The administration of antiviral medications for measles, when deemed necessary, is a decision made in consultation with healthcare providers. Their expertise ensures a thorough assessment of the child's condition, consideration of potential risks, and adherence to established protocols.

It is paramount for caregivers and parents to actively engage in transparent communication with healthcare providers. Understanding the rationale behind the use of antiviral medications, potential side effects, and the expected outcomes contributes to informed decision-making. This collaborative approach ensures that the child receives personalized and attentive care tailored to the unique aspects of their health status.

The landscape of antiviral medications for measles treatment is dynamic, with ongoing research continually shaping our understanding of their role. As scientific inquiry advances, new insights may emerge, leading to refinements in treatment protocols and the development of novel antiviral agents.

Supportive Care and Symptom Relief

Supportive care stands as a cornerstone in the management of measles, emphasizing strategies aimed at sustaining the child's well-being throughout the course of the infection. A pivotal component of supportive care is ensuring adequate hydration, as fever associated with measles can lead to increased fluid loss. Encouraging the child to drink ample fluids, including water and oral rehydration solutions, helps prevent dehydration and maintains overall hydration levels.

Rest assumes a crucial role in the recuperative process. Children with measles often experience fatigue and malaise, necessitating sufficient time for rest and recovery. Creating a comfortable and conducive environment for rest aids in restoring energy levels and supports the body's immune response.

Addressing Fever, Cough, and Other Symptoms: A Targeted Approach

The symptoms accompanying measles, including fever, cough, and other discomforts, can significantly impact the child's quality of life. This chapter outlines a comprehensive strategy for addressing these symptoms, encompassing both pharmacological and non-pharmacological interventions.

Fever Management: Fever-reducing medications, such as acetaminophen or ibuprofen, may be recommended by healthcare providers to alleviate discomfort and control elevated body temperature. It is imperative for caregivers to follow medical guidance meticulously, ensuring proper dosage and adherence to age-appropriate medications. Beyond medication, maintaining a cool and comfortable environment supports the child in managing fever.

Cough Relief: Measles-associated cough can be addressed through a combination of approaches. Humidifiers contribute to moisture in the air, easing respiratory irritation. Warm beverages, such as herbal teas, can provide soothing effects. For children older than one year, honey serves as a natural remedy, known for its cough-suppressant properties. These interventions aim to reduce cough severity and enhance overall respiratory comfort.

Respiratory Hygiene: Maintaining good respiratory hygiene is crucial in preventing secondary infections and minimizing the spread of the virus. Encouraging children to practice proper coughing and sneezing etiquette, disposing of tissues appropriately, and promoting regular hand washing contribute to respiratory health and reduce the risk of additional complications.

In addition, effective implementation of supportive care and symptom relief requires collaboration between caregivers and healthcare providers. Open communication, transparent dialogue about symptoms, and a proactive approach to seeking medical guidance enhance the quality of care provided to the child.

Chapter 6: Bathing an Affected Child with Measles

Gentle Bathing Techniques

Bathing a child affected by measles requires a delicate touch and careful consideration of the sensitivity caused by the measles rash. The need of gentle washing methods as a crucial component of supportive care for the child during their rehabilitation is discussed below.

1. Lukewarm Water and Mild Cleansers

The foundation of gentle bathing lies in choosing the right water temperature and cleansing agents. Lukewarm water is pivotal, as hot water can exacerbate skin irritation. Mild, fragrance-free cleansers should be selected to avoid potential allergens or irritants. The goal is to cleanse the skin gently without causing additional discomfort to the child.

2. Patting Instead of Rubbing

After a thorough cleansing, the child should be dried by patting with a soft towel rather than rubbing. The measles rash can make the skin more sensitive, and a gentle patting motion minimizes friction, reducing the risk of aggravating the rash. This technique helps maintain the cleanliness of the skin while prioritizing the comfort of the affected areas.

3. Special Attention to Rash-Affected Areas

The measles rash tends to concentrate in specific areas, such as the face, neck, and trunk. During bathing, special attention should be given to these rash-affected areas. Gentle strokes and minimal pressure help cleanse the skin without causing undue irritation. The objective is to strike a balance between thorough cleaning and safeguarding the delicate condition of the rash.

4. Adequate Hydration Before Bathing

Ensuring that the child is adequately hydrated before bathing is an additional consideration. Hydration supports the overall well-being of the child and can contribute to the suppleness of the skin. Adequate fluid intake is especially important, as fever associated with measles can lead to increased fluid loss.

5. Choosing Comfortable Bathing Times

Selecting appropriate times for bathing also plays a role in optimizing the child's comfort. Choosing periods when the child is relatively calm and not overly fatigued contributes to a more positive bathing experience. A calm and unrushed atmosphere during bathing enhances the effectiveness of the process.

6. Observing Signs of Discomfort

During the bathing process, caregivers should observe the child for signs of discomfort or distress. If certain areas seem more sensitive, adjustments can be made to minimize contact with those regions. Effective communication with the child, even if they are younger, ensures that the bathing experience is as stress-free as possible.

Using Oatmeal Baths for Skin Relief and Ensuring Comfort and Hygiene

Oatmeal baths have long been recognized for their ability to provide relief from skin irritations, making them a valuable addition to the care routine for a child with measles. The unique properties of oats, including anti-inflammatory compounds, can offer comfort to the child experiencing the discomfort associated with the measles rash.

Preparing an Oatmeal Bath
Creating an oatmeal bath involves incorporating colloidal oatmeal into lukewarm bathwater. Colloidal oatmeal, finely ground oats that readily disperse in water, forms a soothing solution that can be gentle on the child's sensitive skin. Alternatively, placing a cup of regular oats in a muslin cloth and allowing it to steep in the bathwater achieves a similar effect.

Benefits for the Skin
Oatmeal baths are renowned for their ability to alleviate itching, redness, and inflammation associated with skin conditions, including the measles rash. The colloidal oatmeal forms a

protective layer on the skin, assisting in moisture retention and promoting the healing process. This natural remedy not only addresses the physical discomfort but also contributes to the child's overall sense of well-being during a challenging time.

Ensuring Comfort and Hygiene

Selecting appropriate times for bathing is a crucial consideration. Optimal bathing times are when the child is relatively calm and not overly fatigued, ensuring a more positive and soothing experience. Establishing a calm and unrushed atmosphere during bathing contributes to the effectiveness of the process.

Observing Signs of Discomfort

While implementing oatmeal baths, caregivers should keenly observe the child for any signs of discomfort or distress. If certain areas of the skin appear more sensitive, adjustments can be made to minimize contact with those regions. Effective communication with the child, even if they are younger, ensures that the bathing experience remains as stress-free as possible.

Choosing Comfortable Clothing

Post-bath, the choice of clothing becomes crucial in maintaining the child's comfort. Opting for loose-fitting and soft fabrics, particularly cotton, helps prevent unnecessary friction against the measles rash. This choice of clothing contributes to the overall comfort of the child during their recovery.

Hydration and Nutrition

Ensuring that the child remains adequately hydrated is essential for their recovery. Encouraging fluid intake supports overall well-being and helps counteract potential fluid loss associated with fever. A balanced and nutritious diet further contributes to the child's strength and resilience.

While incorporating oatmeal baths and ensuring comfort and hygiene, collaboration with healthcare providers remains pivotal. They can offer personalized recommendations based on the specific condition of the child, the severity of the measles rash, and any additional symptoms present.

Chapter 7: MMR & MMRV Vaccination

Understanding Measles, Mumps, Rubella (MMR) Vaccine: A Tripartite Defense

Composition and Objectives: The MMR vaccine combines weakened or inactivated forms of the measles, mumps, and rubella viruses, triggering an immune response without causing the actual diseases. This trifold defense targets three highly contagious viruses known for their potential to cause severe complications, especially in children.

Measles Component: The measles component of the MMR vaccine is designed to confer immunity against the measles virus. By introducing a harmless version of the virus to the immune system, the vaccine prepares the body to recognize and combat measles, preventing the onset of this infectious disease.

Mumps Component: The mumps component provides protection against mumps, a viral infection characterized by swollen salivary glands. Mumps can lead to complications such as meningitis and deafness, making the inclusion of the mumps component crucial in preventing these potential adverse outcomes.

Rubella Component: Rubella, often milder in children but posing risks during pregnancy, is averted through the rubella component of the MMR vaccine. This ensures that children not only avoid the direct consequences of rubella but also contribute to preventing congenital rubella syndrome in case of pregnancy.

Measles, Mumps, Rubella, Varicella (MMRV) Vaccine

Introduction to MMRV: Building upon the foundation of the MMR vaccine, the MMRV vaccine introduces a fourth component—varicella, commonly known as chickenpox. By combining the protective elements of the MMR vaccine with varicella immunity, the MMRV vaccine provides a comprehensive defense against four viral infections.

Varicella Component: The varicella component addresses the contagious varicella-zoster virus, responsible for chickenpox. Including this in the MMRV vaccine streamlines the vaccination process, offering comprehensive coverage against measles, mumps, rubella, and varicella in a single shot. This not only reduces the number of injections but also enhances the overall convenience of vaccination.

Vaccination Schedule and Importance for Children

Ensuring that children receive timely and appropriate vaccinations is a cornerstone of preventive healthcare. The vaccination schedule, a carefully crafted plan endorsed by healthcare authorities, outlines when children should receive specific vaccines, including the crucial Measles, Mumps, Rubella (MMR) and Measles, Mumps, Rubella, Varicella (MMRV) vaccines. This schedule is designed to maximize the effectiveness of vaccines and provide comprehensive protection during the formative years of a child's life.

Recommended Vaccination Schedule

The vaccination schedule for children is meticulously planned to coincide with critical developmental stages and potential exposure to infectious diseases. The recommended schedule typically begins shortly after birth and extends through adolescence, covering a spectrum of diseases. For MMR and MMRV vaccines, the schedule includes two doses.

1. **First Dose (Around 12-15 Months):** The initial dose of the MMR vaccine is usually administered around 12 to 15 months of age. This timing is strategic, as it ensures that the child receives protection just as the maternal antibodies acquired during pregnancy start to wane. This dose establishes primary immunity against measles, mumps, rubella, and, in the case of MMRV, varicella.

2. **Booster Dose (4-6 Years):** The second dose serves as a booster shot and is typically given between the ages of 4 and 6 years. This reinforces and extends the immune response, providing enduring protection into adolescence and beyond. The MMRV vaccine streamlines this process by incorporating varicella immunity, reducing the number of injections while maintaining comprehensive coverage.

Importance for Children

The importance of adhering to the vaccination schedule for children cannot be overstated. Vaccines, including MMR and MMRV, confer several key benefits:

1. *Disease Prevention*: Vaccines protect children from serious and potentially life-threatening diseases. Measles, mumps, rubella, and varicella can have severe

consequences, especially in younger individuals. Vaccination shields children from the adverse effects of these infections.

2. *Community Immunity*: Following the recommended schedule contributes to the concept of community immunity. When a significant proportion of the population is vaccinated, the spread of infectious diseases is curtailed, protecting those who are unable to receive vaccines due to medical reasons or age. This collective safeguard is crucial for preventing outbreaks.

3. *Long-Term Health:* Vaccinations play a pivotal role in ensuring the long-term health and well-being of children. By preventing the onset of diseases that can have lasting repercussions, such as deafness, encephalitis, or

congenital abnormalities, vaccines contribute to a healthier and more resilient population.

4. *Educational and Social Continuity*: Adherence to the vaccination schedule is often a requirement for enrollment in educational institutions. By ensuring that children receive their vaccinations on time, parents facilitate their educational and social participation without interruptions.

In conclusion, the vaccination schedule for children, including the timely administration of the MMR and MMRV vaccines, is a fundamental aspect of preventive healthcare. Following this schedule not only shields individual children from potentially severe diseases but also contributes to the broader goal of creating healthier and more resilient communities. The importance of vaccination cannot be overstressed, and parents, caregivers, and healthcare providers play pivotal roles in ensuring its successful implementation. They offer personalized guidance, address concerns, and ensure that vaccination decisions align with the child's health status and medical history.

Chapter 8: Spread of Measles among Children

Common Modes of Transmission in Childcare Settings

Airborne Transmission:

Measles is notorious for its airborne transmission, and childcare settings serve as potential hotspots for the spread of the virus. Children, who naturally share spaces in playrooms, classrooms, and other common areas, may unknowingly release infectious respiratory droplets into the air. Coughing, sneezing, or even talking can expel virus-laden particles, creating an environment where susceptible children may inhale the contagion. Proper ventilation and maintaining adequate air quality become pivotal in minimizing the risk of airborne transmission.

Surface Contamination:

Shared surfaces in childcare settings, such as toys, equipment, and furniture, can become fomites for the measles virus. Infected respiratory droplets settle on these surfaces, and unvaccinated or vulnerable children can contract the virus by touching contaminated areas and subsequently touching their face, especially their eyes, nose, or mouth. Regular and thorough disinfection practices, coupled with promoting diligent hand hygiene, are essential in breaking the chain of surface transmission.

Personal Contact:

Children are naturally inclined towards personal contact through play, bonding, and expressions of affection. However, these interactions also create opportunities for the direct spread of measles. Close personal contact, including hugging, holding hands, or playing in close proximity, allows the virus to transfer easily between children. Implementing awareness programs that promote respiratory hygiene and discourage excessive personal contact can be effective in reducing transmission within childcare settings.

Understanding these common modes of transmission within childcare settings is the foundation for designing targeted preventive strategies. By addressing the specific dynamics of measles spread in these environments, caregivers, healthcare professionals, and parents can collaboratively create an environment that minimizes the risk of outbreaks. The subsequent sections of this chapter will explore preventive measures for schools and playgroups and strategies for educating parents and guardians about viral diseases, completing the comprehensive approach to curbing the spread of measles among children.

Preventive Measures for Schools and Playgroups

1. *Vaccination Policies*: The cornerstone of prevention lies in robust vaccination policies within educational settings. Schools and playgroups should enforce stringent policies mandating that all enrolled children are up-to-date with their vaccinations, including the MMR vaccine. By establishing a vaccinated community, the risk of measles transmission is significantly reduced.

2. *Respiratory Hygiene Practices*: Inculcating proper respiratory hygiene practices is

imperative to thwart the spread of measles. Educational institutions should educate children about covering their mouths and noses when coughing or sneezing, using tissues, and disposing of them appropriately. These practices minimize the release of infectious respiratory droplets into the environment.

3. *Frequent Hand Hygiene*: Promoting regular handwashing among children is a fundamental preventive measure. Encouraging proper handwashing with soap and water, especially after using the restroom and before meals, minimizes the risk of transferring the virus from contaminated surfaces to the face. Providing hand sanitizers in strategic locations further supports hand hygiene efforts.

4. *Surface Disinfection*: Regular and thorough disinfection of surfaces, toys, and play

equipment is indispensable. The measles virus can persist on surfaces, posing a continuous threat of transmission. Implementing a routine disinfection schedule using appropriate disinfectants ensures a clean and hygienic environment.

5. *Isolation Protocols*: Institutions should establish clear isolation protocols for children displaying symptoms of measles. The prompt identification and temporary separation of infected individuals prevent the spread of the virus within the educational setting. This proactive approach safeguards the health of other students and staff.

Educating Parents and Guardians about Viral Diseases

1. *Importance of Vaccination*: An informed and supportive parental community is pivotal in the fight against measles. Educating parents about the importance of timely vaccination, specifically the MMR vaccine, is paramount. Clear communication about the vaccine's safety, efficacy, and its role in preventing measles fosters a positive attitude toward immunization.

2. *Recognizing Symptoms:* Parents and guardians should be equipped with the knowledge to recognize early symptoms of measles. A high fever, cough, runny nose, and the characteristic measles rash are red flags that demand immediate medical attention. Prompt identification ensures timely intervention and minimizes the risk of further transmission.

3.   *Transmission   Awareness:*   Creating awareness among parents about the modes of measles transmission enhances their understanding of preventive measures. Emphasizing the highly contagious nature of the virus and the need for vaccination contributes to a collective awareness that supports community immunity.

4. *Community Engagement:* Engaging parents in the educational process fosters a sense of community responsibility. Workshops, information sessions, and community outreach programs provide a platform for open dialogue. This collaborative approach ensures that parents actively participate in preventive measures, creating a resilient and well-informed community.

By implementing these preventive measures in educational settings and actively involving parents in the education process, Chapter 8 aims to create a robust defense against the spread of measles among children. Through a combination of vaccination, hygiene practices, and community engagement, the goal is to establish a health-conscious environment that prioritizes the well-being of every child within the school and playgroup community.

Conclusion: Encouragement for Measles Prevention in Children

Encouragement for Measles Prevention in Children

1. *Celebrating Vaccination Success:* The foundation of measles prevention lies in vaccination, and this chapter celebrates the success stories of widespread immunization. Acknowledging the positive impact of vaccinations on reducing measles incidence and related complications serves as an encouragement to continue and strengthen vaccination efforts.

2. *Empowering Parents and Guardians*: Parents and guardians play a pivotal role in the health of their children. The chapter encourages and empowers parents to prioritize their children's well-being by ensuring timely vaccinations, recognizing early symptoms, and actively participating in preventive measures both at home and within the community.

3. *Highlighting the Resilience of Children*: Children, with their inherent resilience and capacity for recovery, are at the heart of measles prevention. The chapter emphasizes the importance of fostering an environment that nurtures the physical and emotional well-being of children. This includes implementing preventive strategies, promoting healthy habits, and creating supportive communities.

4. *Dispelling Myths and Providing Accurate Information*: Addressing common misconceptions about measles fosters a better understanding of the disease. By dispelling myths and providing evidence-based information, the chapter empowers individuals to make informed decisions about vaccination and preventive measures. Access to accurate information is key to creating a measles-resistant community.

5. *Emphasizing the Role of Community Immunity:* Measles prevention is a collective effort, and the chapter encourages communities to strive for herd immunity. By understanding the significance of community immunity, individuals are motivated to contribute to the overall health of their community. This shared responsibility builds a protective shield against measles outbreaks.

Call to Action: Advocating for Children's Health

1. *Promoting Measles Awareness Campaigns*: The chapter issues a call to action for the initiation and support of measles awareness campaigns. These campaigns serve to educate communities about the importance of vaccination, early symptom recognition, and preventive measures. By leveraging various communication channels, including social media, community events, and educational programs, the call to action aims to reach a wide audience.

2. *Advocating for Accessible Healthcare Services*: Ensuring that healthcare services, including vaccination clinics and educational resources, are accessible to all communities is a

critical aspect of the call to action. Advocacy efforts are directed towards policymakers, healthcare providers, and community leaders to prioritize and enhance healthcare accessibility for children.

3. *Encouraging Research and Innovation:* The call to action extends to the realm of research and innovation. By supporting and advocating for ongoing research into measles prevention, treatment, and the development of advanced vaccines, individuals contribute to the continuous improvement of strategies to protect children from this highly contagious disease.

4. *Creating Supportive Environments*: Advocacy for children's health involves creating environments that prioritize their well-being. This includes safe and hygienic educational

settings, community spaces that facilitate preventive measures, and supportive policies that promote vaccination and health awareness. Advocates are encouraged to collaborate with schools, childcare centers, and local authorities to create such environments.

5. *Fostering Global Collaboration*: The call to action transcends borders, emphasizing the importance of global collaboration in the fight against measles. Advocates are encouraged to support international efforts, contribute to vaccination initiatives in regions with higher prevalence, and engage in partnerships that strengthen the global response to measles.

In conclusion, the final chapter serves as a rallying point for a collective commitment to measles prevention in children. By offering encouragement, dispelling myths, and issuing a compelling call to action, the chapter aims to inspire individuals, communities, and healthcare professionals to actively contribute to the health and well-being of our youngest generation. Measles prevention is not just a medical imperative; it is a shared responsibility and a testament to our commitment to securing a healthy and vibrant future for children worldwide.